MUSTACHE Try-ON Book

By
Hal Malt

Ethos Publishing
Pensacola, Florida

First Printing 2004

Text, Cover design and drawings by Hal Malt
Book edit by Carol Malt, Ph.D.
Production Design by Michael Dawson

ISBN: 0-9714692-2-9
LCCN: 2003091462

ETHOS PUBLISHING
2300 E. Mallory Street, Suite 303
Pensacola. FL 32503

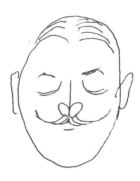

Enjoy
this book or give it to a friend

_ _ _ _ _ _ _ _ _ _ _ _ _ _ _
Feel free to write his name

"What a troublesome, repulsive and ridiculous thing is a mustache; and what a comfort and how irresistible. The mustache is troublesome on a cold and frosty day when your breath freezes and hangs in icicles therefrom. I should think it would be dangerous, as well as troublesome for those who are making their first attempt as I should think it would be apt to destroy their root and branch or do them some serious injury. It is troublesome when eating as your victuals frequently adhere to it. The Mustache is ridiculous when they pretend to have one and are so scattering they are scarcely visible and have to "dye" in order that their mustache may be observed. The mustache is repulsive when besmeared with tobacco juice. On the other hand, the mustache is a great comfort in cold weather in protecting the mouth from the severity of weather. It is also advantageous in hiding any deficiency in the teeth or outline of the mouth. But, oh what an irresistible thing is a soft, silky, waving mustache. I have no words at my command to express my admiration of it so I will leave it for an abler pen."

Alice Stillman, School composition, 1866

INTRODUCTION

Don't face life naked.

Your body provides hair and keeps it coming. What happens to that hair is up to you. This book about facial hair is a handy guide for you to select and enjoy the ideal mustache. Your author has experimented with various mustache designs since urged to grow one eleven years ago. His whiskered appearance on the author's page reflects spouse Carol's guidance in the selection of a more appropriate mustache style.

Maybe a friend lacks a mustache and you would like to offer suggestions. Or you've been mulling the possibility of growing one and been prompted to go ahead and do it. But do what?

On the other hand, if you already have one, perhaps you are ready to change it. You are not quite satisfied. You would rather look more like, well ... picture your favorite role model or actor. You've envied those other men with their dashing look, their masculine presence. You've watched TV, the soaps, wrestling, old movies; riffled magazine pages, oogled mustaches in restaurants and yes, a third or more of the men appeared mustachioed. Theirs seem to come in so many different shapes, sizes and degree of bushiness. You may even have researched library holdings; found that the few references were tomes written by academics for students of hair grooming.

What's more: styles change, you or your partner may have aged or you are bored with the way you look.

Ready for something new and challenging? This book will help you to more easily and quickly experiment. You can see and test various possibilities, visualize which design best suits your face, your desired image, appearance.

Keep this book handy.

"Babies haven't any hair
Old men's words are just as bare
Between the cradle and grave,
Lies a haircut and a shave.
So let's have fun."
Samuel Hoffenstein, 1890-1947

HOW TO USE THIS BOOK

The several chapters contain information on historical styles of facial hair, insights on why many males want mustaches, guidelines for good grooming practice and examples of mustaches for your selection of style. The pages of mustache designs illustrate the more popular ones. Moreover, this book is the first ever to enable you to actually see what each of several possible styles looks like, *on your face*. It answers the question: Which is best for me?

Fifteen styles are provided, each in two sizes in order to relate to faces of different proportion, large or small, as well as different shapes of face, angular or round. We call each design a "Try-ON." Each is easy to cut out and push on using a wad of tape, easy to pull off. So whichever style is first selected, you can easily discard it and try another design. Last but not least, a special page with a grid makes it easy for you to sketch to scale and cutout your own design.

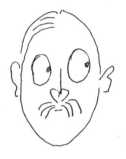

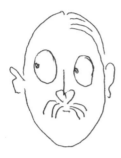

HISTORY ACCORDING to the AUTHOR

About 3000 BC Egyptian men decided to shave their head and face. It was too hot. Plus, being clean-shaven was a sign of nobility. But they were a bit confused because the gods, particularly the Barber God, sported beards. What to do? The elite constructed rectangular beards of clay held onto the chin with string tied around the neck. Even Hatshepsut, a woman who declared herself to be both pharaoh and god and had built an enormous funerary into the side of a cliff, wore a fake beard.

About the same time, Assyrians, who seemed to like their hair dyed red, green or blue and ornamented with gold, rejected mustaches but grew real beards — elegant, fluffy, curled and dyed. On the other hand, Biblical law prohibited Hebrews from cutting their hair so they went about completely whiskered until Delilah cut Samson's hair and he lost his strength.

5

In Classical times, seldom did sculptures or frescoes of Roman heroes display facial hair. And you know what happened to those bare-faced city-builders when the hairy barbarians arrived. As for the Greeks, who admired blond hair, many men and women bleached their dark hair. Men had short hair and kept beards curled in ringlets until Alexander the Great had his troops shaven to avoid having their beards seized in hand-to-hand combat.

Meanwhile, in China and Asia, elders with their droopy mustaches were regarded as paragons of wisdom. Think Confucious. Think Charlie Chan. And look at old prints of mustached Indian nobles — no, not the ones illustrating the many positions of the *Kamasutra*. A bit later, Henry IV, Holy Roman Emperor and King of Germany was excommunicated by Pope Gregory VII because the meat he ate with his fingers gave him greasy whiskers.

Then came the Renaissance. When Anthony Van Dyck painted King Charles I of England with a trim mustache and pointed beard, he created a new style and gained a knighthood. French monarchs and courtiers, the foremost fashion-models for Western Civilization, favored the moustache and flowing locks. Louis XVI wore also a high wig to make him appear taller. At the moment his head was severed by the guillotine, his towering superstructure collapsed as did the cavalier style.

In Russia, when monarch Czar Peter the Great imposed a tax on beards, bristles and tufts of all description disappeared.

Later, in the bustling and burgeoning American colonies, men of affluence displayed facial hair to the extreme as well as wearing white or powdered wigs. So much so that, according to Ripley's Believe It Or Not, it became illegal for a man to wear a beard and mustache. After the Civil War, that law had to be changed because national hero President Ulysses S. Grant demonstrated it was possible to gulp whiskey through whiskers without the aid of a mustache cup. Subsequently most prominent men fostered versions of handlebar 'staches including three other Presidents best left unmentioned.

If the 90's were gay, the Depression of the 30's sent everyone to the movies to see a better life . . . one of sophistication, comedies and musicals. In these, Douglas Fairbanks, William Powell, Don Ameche, Clark Gable and even tough guy James Cagney displayed pencil-thin mustaches. French painter Marcel Duchamp captured that look when he put the mustache on the *Mona Lisa* in the Paris Louvre. Finally even that slight facial adornment had to go. Mothers would now approvingly speak to their daughters of a young man as: "clean cut." Lt. Col. Jacob Schick furthered this image by making shaving easier. In 1926, inspired by his military experience with the army repeating rifle, he invented the Magazine Repeating Razor. This prototype for his injector safety razor used clips easily loaded into the razor.

During this time, women were resorting to many products to enhance their natural beauty. They used corsets, tiny shoes, stiletto heels, bright rouge, hair curlers, the bra. What was available to men? Cologne!

How we've progressed. Women today can more permanently alter their bodies with liposuction, breast implants, tummy tucks and other cosmetic surgery. And so in self-assertion, we now have for men: The Retro Look in Mustache. According to an unscientific poll of young male waiters taken during a Sunday Champagne Brunch at the Pensacola Seville Quarter, the current fashion follows the film star new/old look: two vertical stripes descend from subnasal carpeting to a goatee. Will this contemporary fashion trend last?

And speaking of fashion trends, in what might be the most unusual mustache story to date, numerous stars of stage and screen, female as well as male, sport "Milk Mustaches" in advertisements that promote the beverage. A non-traditional approach to facial enhancement, but one with savvy flair.

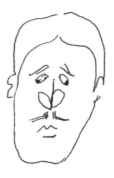

A WORD ABOUT MOTIVATION

Be honest with yourself. You already know that growing and grooming a mustache requires time, patience and enduring a prickly itch while hairs formerly cropped emerge to become stubble. But this initial straggling period of facial hair fortunately is brief, a matter of days. Think why you want to do this. Know that you can achieve the look you seek and admire. And don't be afraid to try out different styles — no mustache is permanent. Even if you do nothing, do not trim, it will change from day to day. Above all, relax and enjoy the process. It's not often men can play with what nature has given them.

Here Are Eleven Common Reasons to Grow and Nurture Facial Hair

- be macho, not a wimp, be distinctive
- make women swoon
- significant other likes it
- big screen idol wears one
- make my baby face look older
- make my wrinkled face look younger
- accent the positive, minimize the negative
- it's the only thing I can change about me
- I can always shave it off
- for the hell of it

Consider the above listing. Each selected reason has both implications and consequences. Regard the first item: "be distinctive." That means stand out, be different. But appear notable in what manner? Do you want a Cool Look? He-man? Sophisticated? Portrayed to what degree?

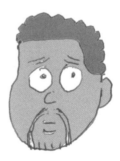

WORK WITH WHAT YOU HAVE

All walruses have large mustaches of especially sensitive whiskers that help them detect food on the dark sea floor. With humans, a walrus mustache is a "crumb catcher." Large whiskers and food are not necessarily compatible. What's more, no two faces are exactly alike. If this weren't so, think how difficult criminal identification would be. Or, on an equally dubious note, all women would fall in love with that one male face — everyone's ideal.

In general, there are three approaches to creating a mustache that will determine your facial appearance.

- ✓ Follow your facial characteristics
- ✓ Express personality — yours or wannabe
- ✓ Go with the latest fad

Are your facial features large or small? Look at your eyes. Are they your best facial feature? If so, don't sport an unusual or very large mustache that will compete with or minimize that noteworthy feature.

Does the nose come down close to the upper lip? That facial area between, according to Jack Kichler, MD and Dermatologist, is known as "supralabial." Examine that space between nose and upper lip. Does it seem large or small? Do you want to completely cover it with hair or not?

Then too, many of us have a slight depression in the upper lip, some a very pronounced one. Those admired film stars of the thirties and forties — Clark Gable for example — emphasized that feature. He split the mustache in two, leaving a wide space between the thin halves, a part in the facial hair, so to speak. If that's your look, leave the gap, shave the two halves to a narrow line and you're in like Flynn.

Is the nose with nostrils, broad or slender? What about the nasolabial fold, those under-cheek grooves, slight or deep, that angle from the top of the nostril to the corner of the mouth? Is that a geometry to be respected or ignored?

Harmony is what you are looking for. That means the mustache should work with your facial features. Unless the intent is to call attention at any cost, the mustache should be proportionate to the face. Hitler had a distinctive mustache. His was very tall and narrow but full. Made him look like a pipsqueak until we learned better. Comedians Charlie Chaplin and Oliver Hardy wore similar mustaches. Made the skinny one look pathetic and the fat one funny.

The goal might be to achieve your own identity. Have the mustache say who you are. Once you find your look, keep it.

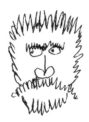

WHAT TYPE HAIR HAVE YOU

First, consider some hair characteristics. We humans must make do with the quantity of active hair follicles on the head we are born with. That quantity diminishes with age. Scalp hair shedding differs between people; a loss of up to 100 hairs a day is normal. Fortunately hair loss on the face is less. The follicles (which contain root and bulb beneath the skin) do not disappear from the face as fast as those on the top of the head. Your face has about 15,000 whiskers. On average, hair grows about one half inch a month with fine hair (light color) a little less, while coarse hair (dark color) grows a bit more and faster.

When you first let the facial hair grow — don't despair. Hairs will stick straight out. They will not brush or shape in the direction you want. Everyone experiences this, unless all you have is "peach fuzz." If you are looking to sprout a handlebar mustache, be patient. Give it another week or more.

Some academic books classify the human hair types into as many as eight different categories. (The editor advises: "That's splitting hairs.") Here we only distinguish between three major types: straight, wavy or kinky. One type will likely be more amenable to one style of mustache design than will another. For example, kinky hair tends to stick outward from the face . . . kinky hairs projecting from the upper lip in a thin line will look a bit strange. Straight hairs can more readily be trained to lay flat and parallel. Your hair type is one of the considerations influencing choice of the style to grow and nurture.

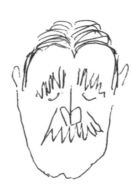

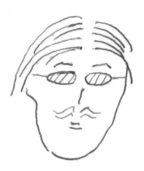

GROOM for the BRIDE

Hair Coloring

To do or not to do. This is not as ridiculous as it may sound. Facial hair on some men appears as a different color than hair on the scalp or sides of the head. Your author's mustache came in red in contrast to the black hair on the sides. (Don't ask about the sparse top.) Then too, the mustache may show gray before other areas of the head do, which some believe creates a distinguished look.

Changing hair color is big business in the United States and abroad, for men as well as women. In Eastern Europe and Russia, at this time, pink hair color is popular.

Many consumer product companies use strong chemical products to make changes in the natural color of hair. Over time the chemicals may damage hair or skin, not to mention maintenance becoming a nuisance. But you won't convince the millions of women who use hair-coloring products to stop. You could try shoe polish which has a distinctive male odor. But be aware it is toxic and may have social consequences.

Shampoo

When you shampoo your head you might as well do the mustache too. Cleansing will remove dirt and oils from skin and hair shafts. Also, your local supermarket may stock a loofah, a sponge-like gourd that effectively removes dead skin cells.

To tell when your hair is clean, grasp fingerfulls of hair and gently pull. Clean hairs should squeak. Shampoos are available that promise to medicate, shine, volumize, moisturize and revitalize. Snake oil is not desirable. Nor is an alkaline product. A mild, low pH shampoo will not harm hair follicles.

Bush Pruning Tools

Your choice is threefold: straight-blade, trimmer or scissors. There are proponents for each. You are wise enough not to try chemical depilation.

A stickler for tradition will be a wet blade shaver and get a shave closer to the skin plus a bloody nick here or there but that's what styptic pencils are for. Outside the bathroom, do not use toilet paper on the wound. After three shaves throw away your single-edge razor, that's why you buy a bag full.

Washing your face with warm water just before shaving softens and opens the pores helping reduce cuts. It is not necessary to put a steaming cloth over your face as do barbers prior to shaving, but you will sigh with pleasure if you do.

Trimmer

Try wet shaving in - 40° Fahrenheit weather.

Electric razors now are technological marvels. Multiple blades oscillate beneath perforated foils. Norelco has several unique models with floating heads that hug facial contours. Compare brands and prices at DealTime on the Internet.

A visit to your local pharmacy or discount store is instructive. Shelves are lined with clear plastic boxes displaying a multitude of electric razors at prices upward of $9.99. Many are packaged as kits with cleaning brush, mustache comb and attachments including nose, ear and eyebrow clipper. Designs frequently change. Innovations occur such as self-cleansing and vacuum collection of hair clippings. Each company may produce several models. Read the fine print on the packages and compare.

Most electric shavers require the skin to be dry for use. A five-star Norelco model moisturizes as it cuts. If you travel, make sure yours is cordless and rechargeable.

Scissors

Do not use household scissors — they are difficult to control and their sharp points stab and scratch. Barbers' scissors have rounded points as well as a spur or tang which helps the little finger brace or stabilize the instrument. Professionals, when "edge-cutting," comb the hair down; the thumb holds the bottom blade to the face and that blade's flat edge is slid under the hairs along the upper lip. The little and next finger actuate the top blade which should make small one half inch snips. The cutting blade has tiny serrations that keep hair groups from sliding away.

A source for professional 5 inch stainless steel scissors is: Bob Ohnstad (a practicing barber), Home Haircutter's Supply, P.O. Box 11400, Minneapolis, Minnesota 55411.

Waxing

Your author twirls both ends of his modified Royal Air Force mustache without wax. For those who don't care to act and look like the villain in *The Perils of Pauline*, wax is your alternative. Speaking of which, you again have choices: stiff wax or soft. Do not use ski wax! Use a product from Clubman.

If you are striving for pointed ends or working on a large handlebar that you want to curl up from the lip —but perhaps it is unruly — you want the stiff wax. Its use takes considerable technique but experiments can be washed out easily with hot water and shampoo. Starting with a dollop the size of a pea on your finger, apply it to the middle of your damp 'stache. Use a comb to spread it through the hairs adding more wax every half inch. Give it an approximate shape with your fingers then stop. Twist the hairs at the end a bit to get them together and the others parallel to each other. Wait several minutes until the wax has dried and stiffened. Now use your fingers to give it the final shape desired. (Don't try to comb. In this hardened state, you'll pull out hairs.)

If your hair seems pliable or you want your mustache to be a droopy western style, you could use the soft wax. It is not necessary to sleep with a bandana wrapped around your head and waxed mustache as did Hercule Poirot in *Death on the Nile*. And remember when waxed not to lean over a candle or go sunning at the beach unless you are under an umbrella.

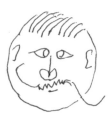

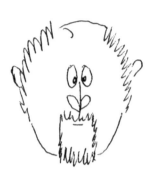

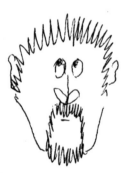

USING Try-ON

Experimenting with Try-ON is quick and easy.

The photographs on the next page illustrate experiments with five mustache styles. In this simple procedure, the model shown below made a selection from the fifteen examples depicted in the second half of the book and cut them out. Next, a small strip of masking tape was folded and adhered to the back of each shape. Voila! The fun and laughter began.

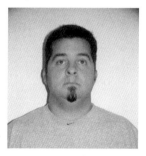

21

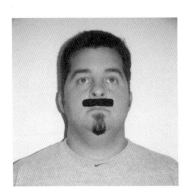

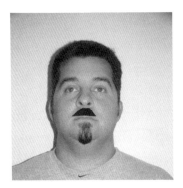

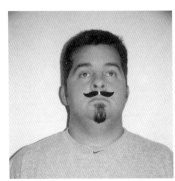

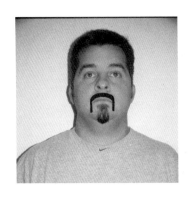

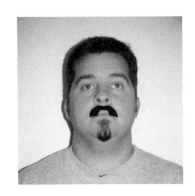

15 STYLES TO CUTOUT AND TRY

Why so many choices?

Unlike male clothing that changes little from year to year, the favored mustache design de jour may change as fast as the MTV or Hollywood "look" of the year. Over a recent short period, celebrity fashion changed from mustache over a clean-shaven chin, to "soul" patch on the chin, to mustache descending and merging with a larger patch known as a goatee. Multiple style choices are here presented to help you find that one image most comfortable and appropriate. Fifteen designs are each presented in two sizes to better serve differing facial characteristics. That is, the top version on a page is intended to be suitable for a smaller or thinner face and the bottom mustache for a larger or rounder face.

If this is a library copy, please do not cut out any mustache drawings. Copy them instead.

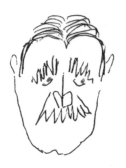

BOOMERANG

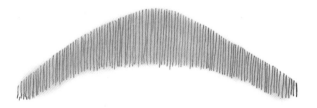

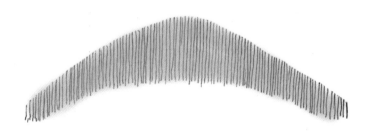

This page intentionally left blank.

RHETT BUTLER

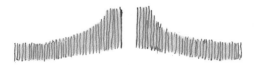

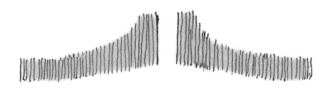

This page intentionally left blank.

COWBOY

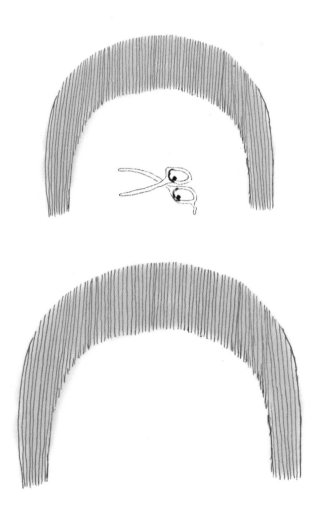

This page intentionally left blank.

THE OFFICE

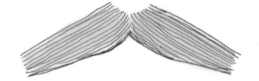

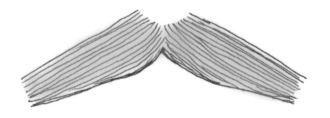

This page intentionally left blank.

HANDLEBAR

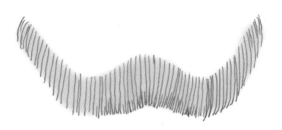

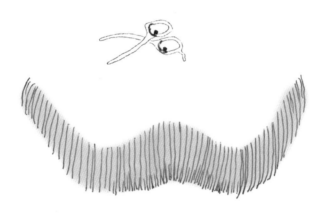

33

This page intentionally left blank.

BELGIAN DETECTIVE

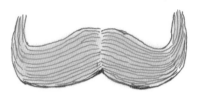

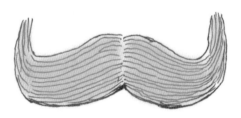

This page intentionally left blank.

FU MANCHU

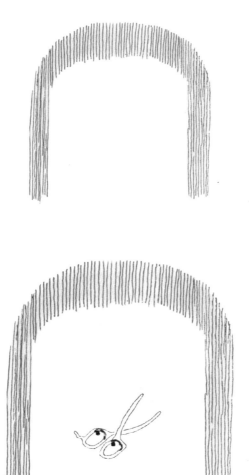

This page intentionally left blank.

MILITARY

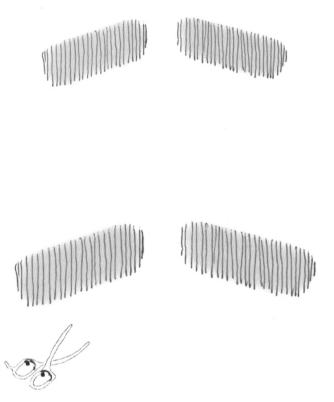

This page intentionally left blank.

PAINT BRUSH

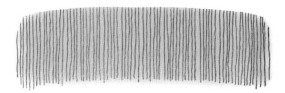

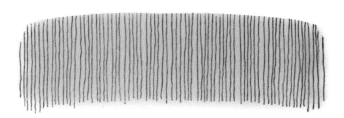

41

This page intentionally left blank.

ROLLER COASTER

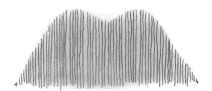

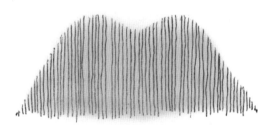

43

This page intentionally left blank.

BARBER SHOP

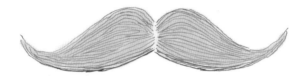

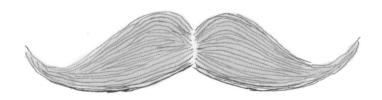

This page intentionally left blank.

STIFF UPPER LIP

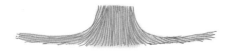

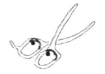

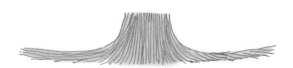

This page intentionally left blank.

WALRUS

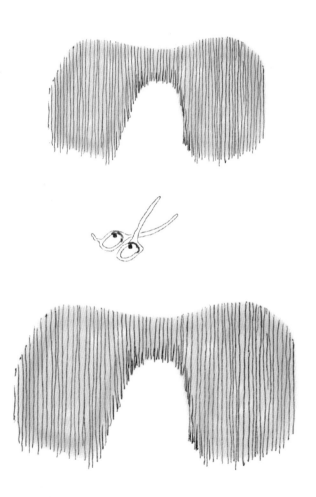

This page intentionally left blank.

BARBELL

51

This page intentionally left blank.

FLAIR

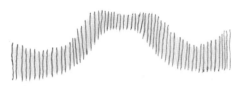

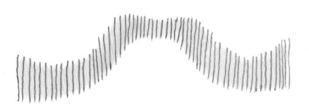

This page intentionally left blank.

Create Your Own Style

You did not find one of the given styles to be exactly right? Perhaps it didn't quite match the vision of yourself you had in mind? sketch your own style then cutout your design. Each page has a 1/4 grid providing a sense of scale and symmetry as you draw. You can even color it with crayons or markers.

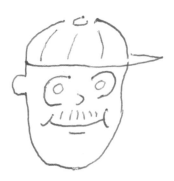

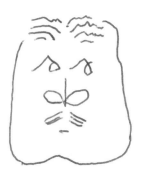

SKETCH GRID

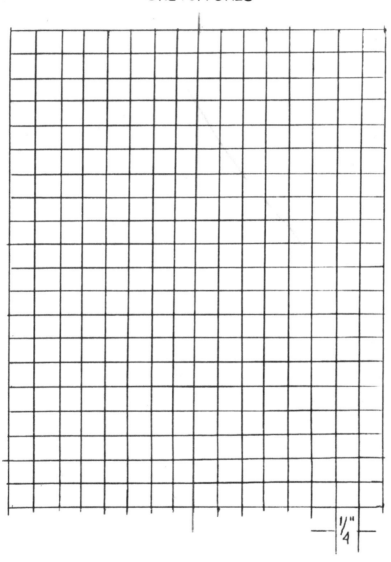

¹/₄"

ABOUT THE AUTHOR

MUSTACHE Try-ON BOOK
ISBN: 0-9714692-2-9

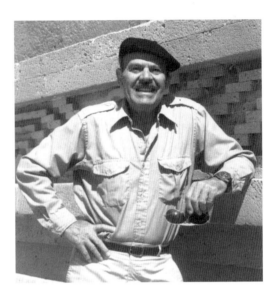

Hal Malt in the ruins of Monte Alban, Oaxaca, Mexico

Hal Malt, author of the Mustache Try-On Book, is an industrial designer, urban designer, University of Miami Professor Emeritus of Architecture and Urban Planning, writer of academic books and a pilot. He created this personalized book for every man who wants style...every woman who appreciates a masculine face.

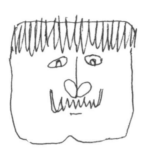